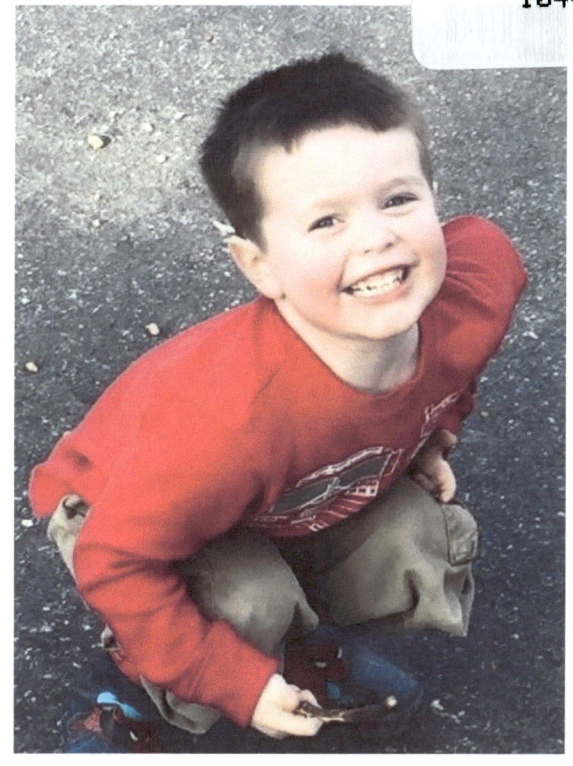

I Am Jake

I have brown hair,

blue eyes, and

T1D

by Natalie Fisher Guerin

I Am Jake

I have brown hair,
blue eyes, and
T1D

by Natalie Fisher Guerin

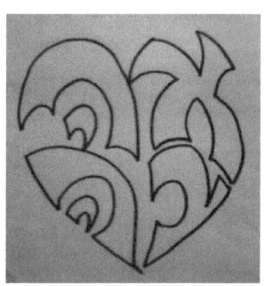

This book is dedicated to my grandson,

Jacob,

who is a light in my life -

and the only one

in my family

who likes me to sing to him.

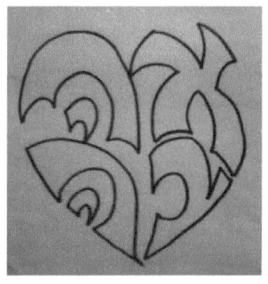

This book is dedicated to my grandson,

Jacob,

who is a light in my life -

and the only one

in my family

who likes me to sing to him.

I am Jake.

I'm three years old.

When I was only fifteen months old, we got on a very big airplane and flew for a long time to visit some of my family.

It was a lot of fun playing with my cousins.

But then I started feeling really tired and didn't want to play.

I didn't even want to eat.

I was so thirsty! I just kept drinking more water and more water.

And Mom had to change my diaper every hour.

My Mom got worried.

She took me to urgent care.

The doctor said I had an ear infection.

Mom knew that being very, very thirsty is a sign of diabetes so she asked the doctor who told her that I was too young to have diabetes, that children don't get diabetes until around seven years old.

The doctor was wrong.

Two days later I was so sick that I couldn't even lift up my head.

All I could do was cry for more water to drink.

Mom took me to the hospital. They took some blood and tested it.

That's when the doctor told my Mom that I did have diabetes.

I didn't know what that word meant but I do now.

They even put a needle into me that stayed in me.

It's called an "IV".

I had never heard that word before either but it's a way to get stuff inside of you.

They put me and Mom in an ambulance and sent us to another hospital that was especially for kids.

They even called it a "children's hospital".

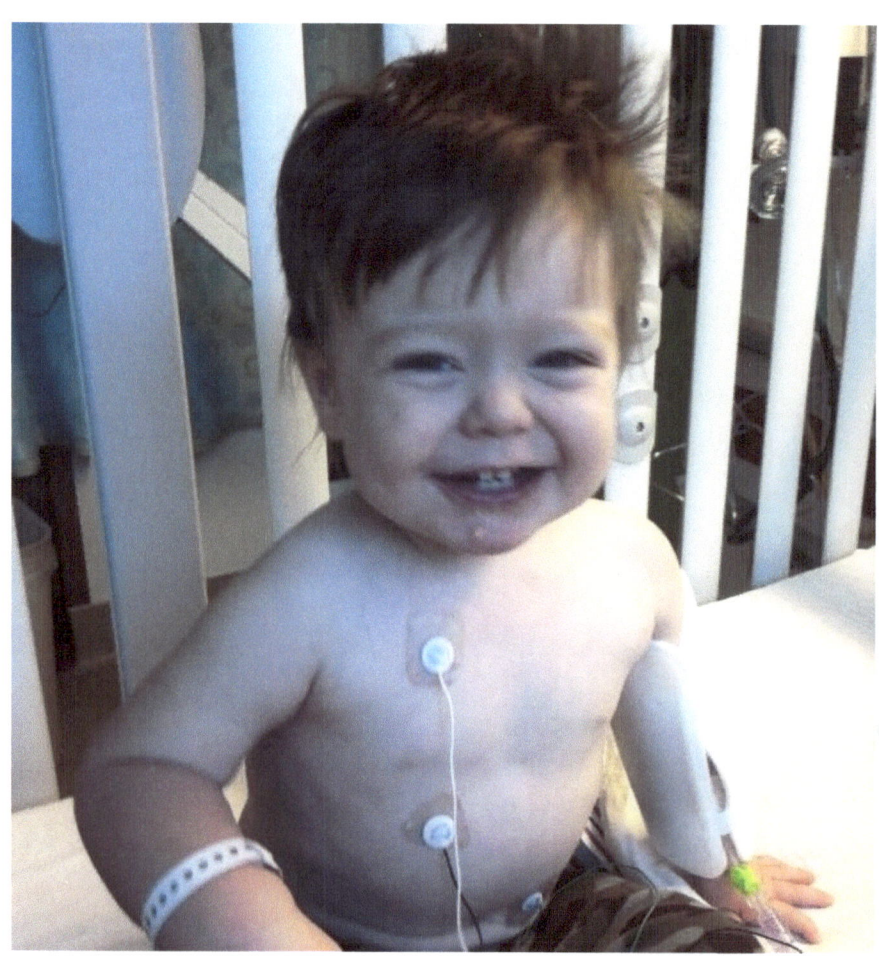

I was feeling so sick but once the IV started working, I felt much better.

I stayed in the hospital until they knew I was okay.

And my Mom had to learn how to take care of me.

After a few days, we got to fly back home.

I was really happy to be back in my own house.

I had missed my Dad, my dog and all of my toys.

My Mom, Dad, brother, Grammy and I all went to meet my new special diabetes doctor and his nurse.

Both of them also have diabetes.

The nurse taught my Dad and Grammy how to prick my finger so they could get a drop of blood and put it on a special piece of paper that goes into a little machine.

When they do it, the machine shows a number, called my "blood sugar number".

They want the number to be between 100 and 200.

My family learned what to do if the number is too low or too high.

When Mom first took me to the hospital, my number was over 900.

I was feeling so sick but once the IV started working, I felt much better.

I stayed in the hospital until they knew I was okay.

And my Mom had to learn how to take care of me.

After a few days, we got to fly back home.

I was really happy to be back in my own house.

I had missed my Dad, my dog and all of my toys.

My Mom, Dad, brother, Grammy and I all went to meet my new special diabetes doctor and his nurse.

Both of them also have diabetes.

The nurse taught my Dad and Grammy how to prick my finger so they could get a drop of blood and put it on a special piece of paper that goes into a little machine.

When they do it, the machine shows a number, called my "blood sugar number".

They want the number to be between 100 and 200.

My family learned what to do if the number is too low or too high.

When Mom first took me to the hospital, my number was over 900.

The doctor said that often a child goes into a coma before the parents realize something is wrong.

It doesn't hurt too much when they prick my finger.

It's something they have to do.

They ask me which finger to use and I get to choose. I like that part.

The nurse also taught them how to give me a shot.

Sometimes they do that when I'm playing so I don't notice it too much.

I know they have to do these things because they love me and want to take care of me.

While they were learning all of this, my brother Gabe and I got to play with our toys on the floor.

I didn't really understand all the words the doctor and nurse were saying in the beginning but now I do.

When you have diabetes, it means that your pancreas doesn't work right.

Your pancreas is something inside of you.

What's supposed to happen is that, when you eat, your pancreas releases something called insulin which changes the food so that your body can use it.

If your pancreas doesn't work right, and no insulin is released, you have to get the insulin from a shot.

Right now an adult gives me shots during the day for the food I eat.

When I get old enough, I will learn how to give myself the shots.

My doctor and nurse gave my family lots to read so they could learn about diabetes.

Food has something called "carbs" in it.

Carbs make my number go up.

So, the adult who gives me food needs to know how many carbs are in it so they know how much insulin to give me in my shot.

Some foods are called "carb free" and I can eat them without needing a shot.

Some foods have a lot of carbs in them so, if I eat them, I might need another shot.

I'm learning what foods can mean I might need an extra shot, foods like candy, cake and ice cream.

But that's okay.

It means I can have whatever the other kids are having, like at a birthday party.

One day, after I had my shot for what I ate for lunch, my number kept going higher.

My Mom called the doctor's special phone and left a message.

She was getting ready to take me to the hospital when the doctor called her back.

He said that the insulin may have gone bad, to throw it out and to give me another shot.

He was right. The second shot worked and I felt a lot better.

Sometimes, when people learn that I have diabetes, they think that I'm a sick kid.

I am not a sick kid.

I can do anything that any other kid can do.

My Dad built us a tree house with a climbing wall.

I really like to play in that.

I also like to play soccer, shoot hoops, ride my bike, and play with my dog.

We live near the water and I really like to go there.

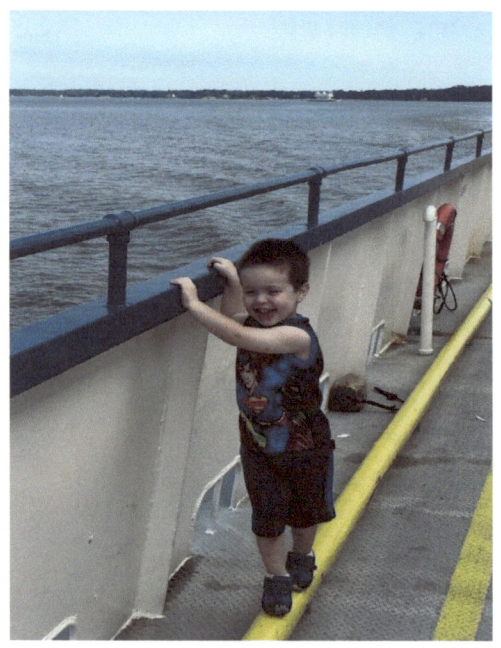

We have a trampoline in the back yard that's a lot of fun.

She was getting ready to take me to the hospital when the doctor called her back.

He said that the insulin may have gone bad, to throw it out and to give me another shot.

He was right. The second shot worked and I felt a lot better.

Sometimes, when people learn that I have diabetes, they think that I'm a sick kid.

I am not a sick kid.

I can do anything that any other kid can do.

My Dad built us a tree house with a climbing wall.

I really like to play in that.

I also like to play soccer, shoot hoops, ride my bike, and play with my dog.

We live near the water and I really like to go there.

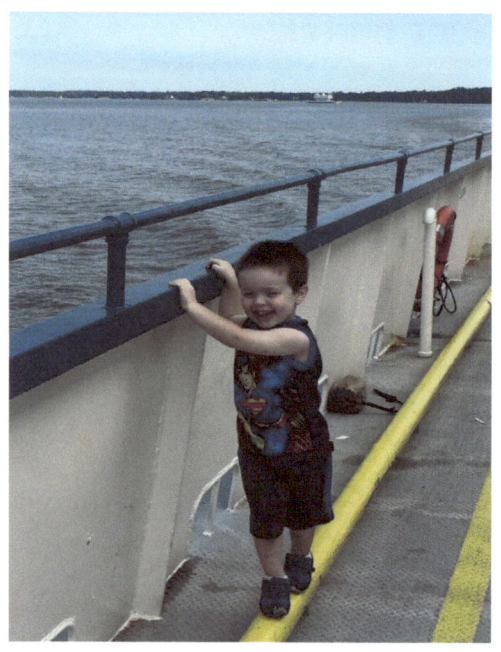

We have a trampoline in the back yard that's a lot of fun.

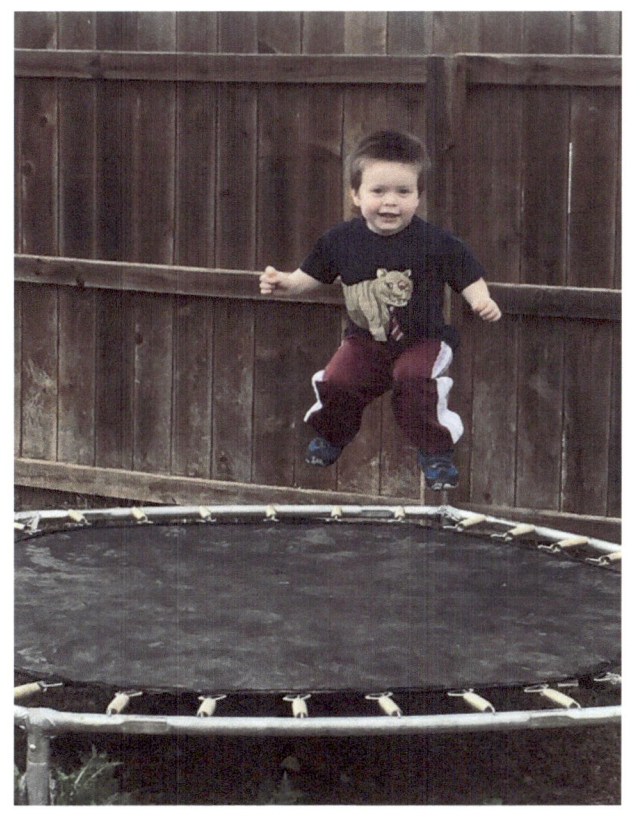

I'm in preschool.

My teachers had never had a diabetic kid before - that's what they call a kid with diabetes - a diabetic kid.

The people in charge of the school told my Mom she had to stay on the school grounds in case they needed her - until my teachers could meet with my doctor's nurse to learn what they needed to learn.

Even teachers need to learn new stuff!

Once they learned about diabetes, they felt better knowing they could take good care of me.

I am happy when it's a school day. I get to play with all of my new friends. We do lots of fun things.

I even learned to play the guitar.

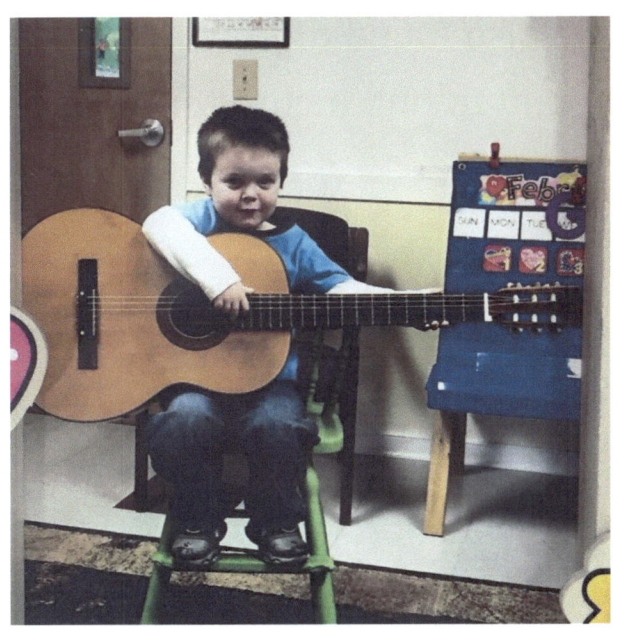

When my Mom first found out I had diabetes, she started a playgroup for me with other kids who have diabetes.

I was glad to know I wasn't the only one.

She also found a group of people who are working to find a cure for diabetes. It's called JDRF.

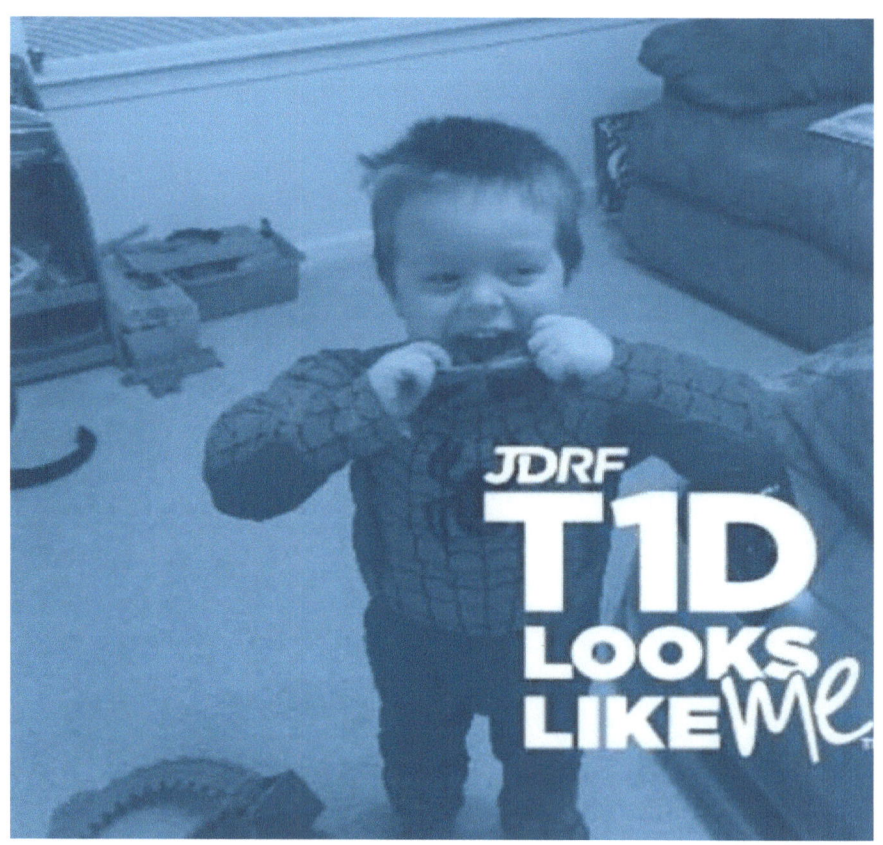

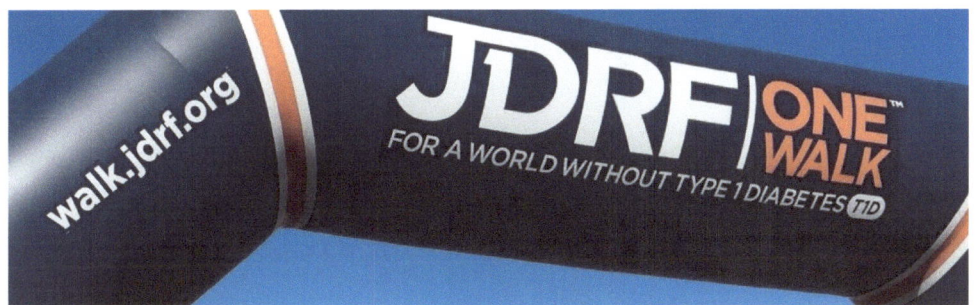

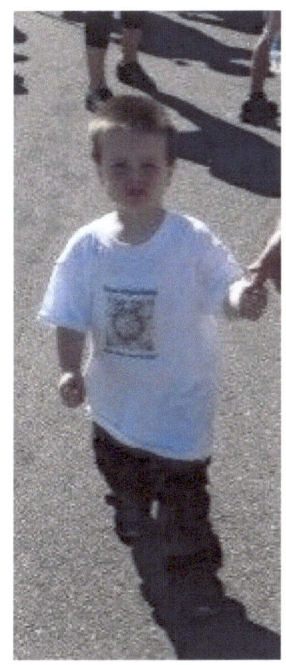

Sometimes the people at JDRF pick a day and a whole bunch of people come and march together. They call it the "Walk for the Cure". The first time a lot of my Mom and Dad's friends came to the march and they called us "Team Sugarbaby". My Mom brought a stroller for me but I wanted to walk.

There's a lot I'll have to learn about my diabetes as I get older so that I can take care of myself.

Even now, I have to learn the signals of being high or low so I can tell Mom and Dad and they can help me.

I've learned that I'm lucky to live in a time when they have insulin because I can do anything that any other kid can do.

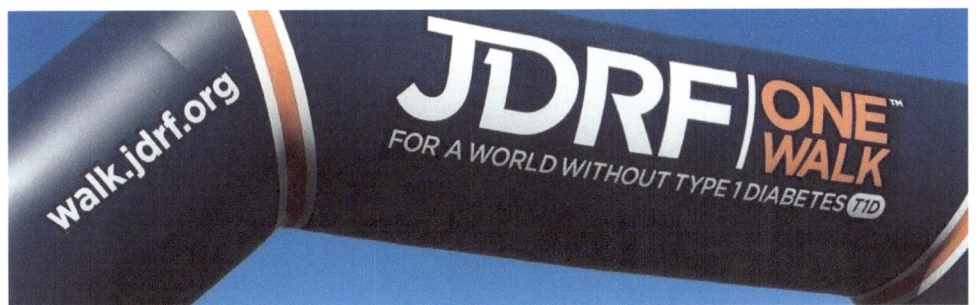

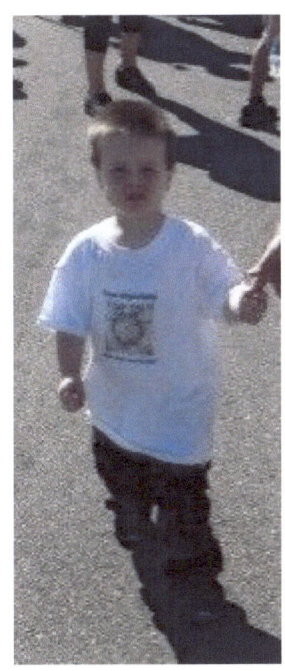

Sometimes the people at JDRF pick a day and a whole bunch of people come and march together. They call it the "Walk for the Cure". The first time a lot of my Mom and Dad's friends came to the march and they called us "Team Sugarbaby". My Mom brought a stroller for me but I wanted to walk.

There's a lot I'll have to learn about my diabetes as I get older so that I can take care of myself.

Even now, I have to learn the signals of being high or low so I can tell Mom and Dad and they can help me.

I've learned that I'm lucky to live in a time when they have insulin because I can do anything that any other kid can do.

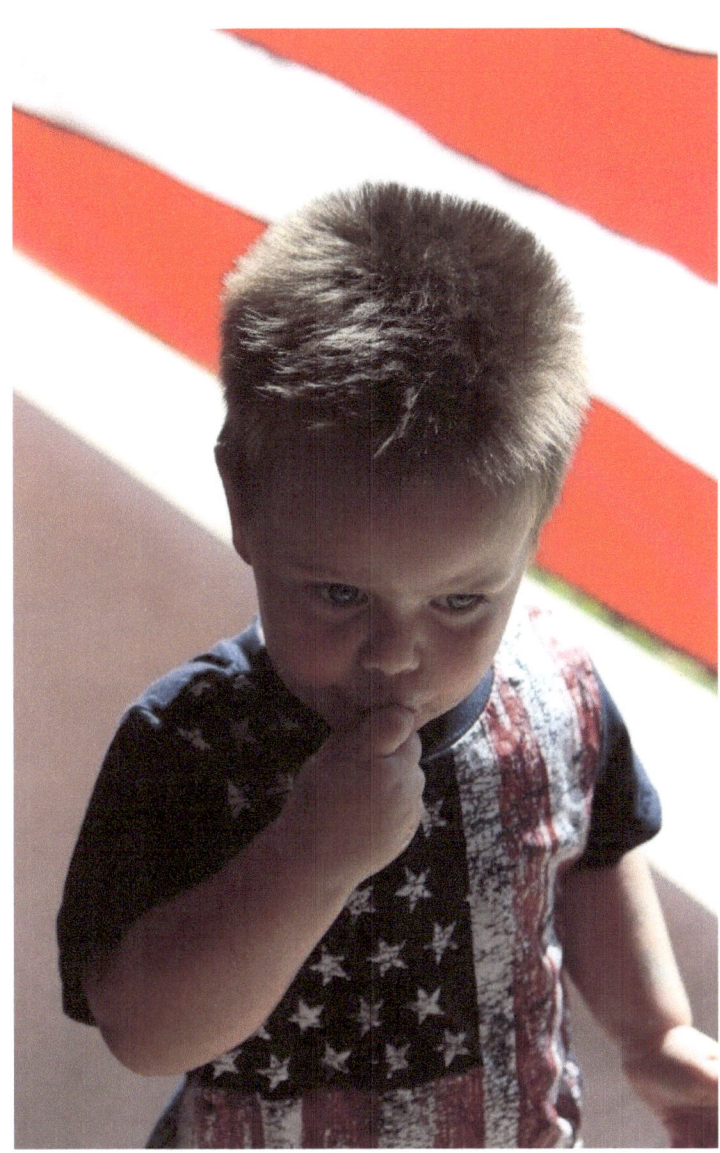

I Am
Jake

I have
brown
hair,
blue
eyes,
and
T1D

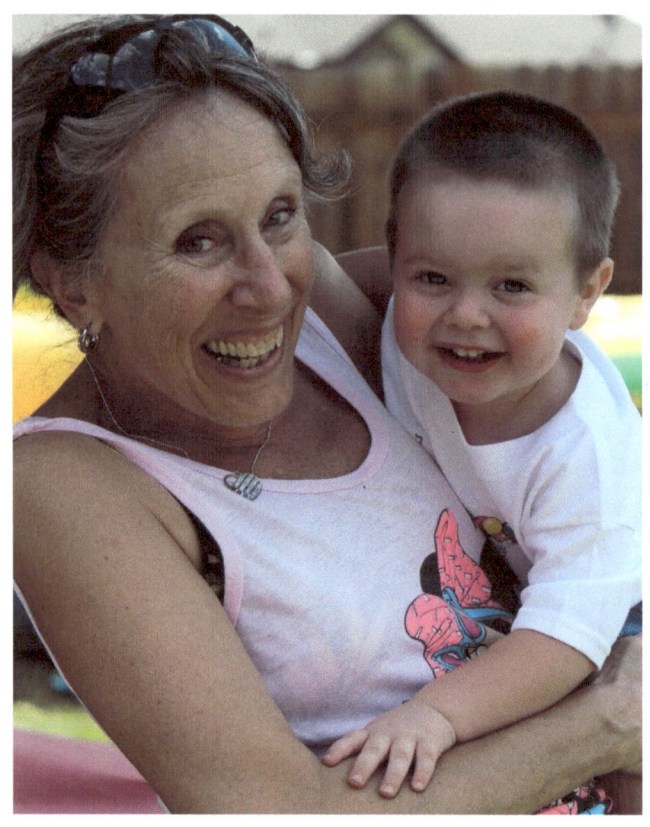

Natalie Fisher Guerin with then two-year-old Jake, who was diagnosed with Type One Diabetes (T1D) at the age of 15 months.

It is her hope that this book will help families who have just learned that their child has this auto-immune disorder.

She previously wrote "Always, a love story between you and your child" and "One Way Ticket to Kona", which are available at www.AttiePublishing.com